Gout Demystified

A Simplified Approach to Neutralize
Hyperuricemia

Hemen Ee

2015

Contents

Introduction

This book is neither fiction nor scientific. I am writing this to share my rather unconventional understanding of gout based on my experience with thousands of gout patients. I would like to clarify that I'm not a doctor or any medical professional. The information shared in this book is for the purpose of enriching your understanding of gout from a different perspective.

I do not have high uric acid and have never experienced any gout attack at all. It was a rather adventurous journey of how I ended up becoming a "gout expert" to the extent that some of my clients regard me as more "doctor" than the doctors who failed to solve their gout miseries.

It all started eight years ago when I was the marketing manager of a company promoting an alkaline water ionizer. Instead of focusing on selling the technical features of the water ionizer, I was more intrigued by what kind of modern diseases could be cured by drinking ionized alkaline water. I read many books about the importance of body pH and how acidosis has led to the onset of a global epidemic of health crises. Out of so many modern diseases, gout caught my attention because my then 60-year-old father was suffering from it. His blood uric acid level was above healthy range for many years, and he was complaining about having joint pains whenever he ate too much meat or drank too much beer.

I did some research online and realized that gout is actually not really as complicated as many people think it is. It is a condition where the excess uric acid in the body reaches the saturation point and crystalizes near the joints. The body perceives these fine urate crystals as foreign invaders and alerts the body's immune system to trigger the very painful gouty inflammation.

Once I got the picture clear, my simple logical, scientific mind concluded that ionized alkaline water could definitely help my dad lower his uric acid level and eventually stop the painful gout attacks once and for all.

Simple science explains it all. The pain is triggered by the urate crystals. The crystals are from the excess uric acid. The only thing on earth than can neutralize acid is alkaline.

A few months after I had installed a unit of alkaline water ionizer in my parents' house, my father went for his yearly body checkup. The blood test report showed that his blood uric acid level was back to the healthy range. This has convinced me that ionized alkaline water is very effective in reducing the blood uric acid level and preventing gout attacks.

From then on, gout became my most effective marketing keyword. In all marketing events, we focus on looking for people troubled by gout, and we even guaranteed the prospect that a person's blood uric acid level will drop significantly within three months if he drinks ionized alkaline water frequently.

After seeing enough successful cases, I am so sure about the result that I can even personally provide a money-back guarantee. If the blood uric acid level or gout attack frequency doesn't drop after three months of drinking ionized alkaline water, I will refund the full amount paid by the client. Until today, I have never received any request for a refund.

As our sales increased, so did my confidence in ionized alkaline water. I extended my scope of research further to other diseases while looking for ways to reach out for more gout patients to show them the new effective approach of getting rid of gout. I realized I could reach only a very small percentage of gout patients through conventional marketing channels, usually road shows and limited advertising.

I could not print any flyer or brochure with a headline like "Ionized Water Can Cure Gout" or any other implicit way of expressing that message. The use of disease names in any form of commercial advertisement is regulated by the health ministry. It is very hard to convince the group of highly educated bureaucrats that something as simple as water can be the ultimate cure for gout. Eventually, I learned that the modern medical industry is dominated by Big Pharma. They have the power to lobby the politicians so that related laws are enacted in favor of their business.

Big Pharma controls the media and indirectly "educates" the doctors and the policymakers. As soon as they enter medical school, doctors are trained to use medicines and surgeries to treat illnesses. Under the influences of various forms of media publicity, modern society is programmed to believe that a person wearing a white coat with a stethoscope hanging around her neck is the only official life savior. We have also been brainwashed to believe that the expensive medicines and advanced medical devices are created to save us. Welcome to the era of medical industrialization!

It is not the objective of this book to discuss the problems of a modern corrupted health care system. If you are interested in this topic, you can Google it yourself.

Let's get back to the main topic of this book: how to get rid of gout permanently. I urge you to keep an open mind as you read through this book. By the time you finish reading this book, I am sure you will be delighted to know that gout can be cured completely.

Chapter 1

Why Doctors Have Failed to Get Rid of Your Gout

Still remember the very first time you experienced a gout attack? Gout usually flares up early in the morning. Most probably, your first gout pain hit you when you were sleeping soundly. Suddenly, you were awakened by the intense pain in your foot, a sensation similar to a sprained joint. While trying to recall when and where did you kick a hard stone, the swollen joints seemed to grow larger and more painful.

You hopped your way to look for aspirin hoping that it would take away the unbearable pain. A few hours after you have popped in the pill, it seemed as though it was not working in reducing the pain and inflammation. You started to worry, wonder if there is any bone fracture due to sleepwalking since you couldn't recall kicking anything hard yesterday.

Eventually, you ended up in the clinic to seek answers and solutions from your respected doctor. As soon as the doctor saw the way you hopped into the room and looked at the red swollen joint, without the need of an X-ray, your doctor said, "Oh! That's gout!" And then the doctor asked what did you eat the last few days and gave you some brief explanation and advice on gout. He prescribed colchicine and painkiller for you. You took the pills as instructed and gout disappeared in a few days. You thought it was cured.

After a few months, your second gout attack visited. You visited your doctor again, listened to the same old consultation, and took the pills. Gout disappeared after a few days. Another few months passed by, and your third gouty inflammation attacked. This cycle repeated again and again, and a "holiday" duration between attacks became shorter and shorter, from months to weeks. Eventually, you got fed up with the doctor and here you are, reading this book.

Does This Conversation Sound Familiar to You?

Gout patient: Doc, why can't my gout problem go away even though I've followed your instruction and finished the whole course of medication?

Doctor: Oh, you have to understand that gout cannot be cured; you have to live with it for the rest of your life. Those medications can only help in reducing your pain and regulating the purine and uric acid level in your blood.

Gout patient: You mean I'll have to go for medical consultation and blood tests every month and continue buying those drugs for the rest of my life?

Doctor: Yup. I'm sorry to tell you that you have no other option.

Gout patient: You mean I have to continue wasting money on those drugs even though it's proven that it will never cure my gout problem?

Doctor: That's a hard sad fact of life.

Gout patient: What?!

The fact is those medications not only cannot get rid of the accumulated uric acid but also indirectly increase other acidic toxic compounds in your body over the years. This is because almost all drugs are acidic or toxic, which eventually leads to secondary illnesses, such as hypertension, diabetes, or kidney failure.

This path of treating gout is heading toward a dead end. Eventually, you will die because of either kidney failure or liver failure due to overconsumption of NSAIDs or steroidal painkillers, in the form of either oral pills or injections. You must look for other ways out before it is too late.

If you Google "alternative gout cure" or "natural remedies for gout," most probably you will get such answers as baking soda, apple cider vinegar, cherries, or some traditional herbs. The fact is that the alternative medicine world still does not have any solid logical and proven effective solution for gout either. This has left many gout patients in constant despair and helplessness.

The sad fact is that neither your doctor nor your homeopathist can free you from the torture of gout attacks. The approach of using prescription drugs or natural herbs to cure gout has failed. They can only manage the pain but not get rid of the root of gout, the uric acid.

Forget what you've learned about gout before this. If it had worked, you wouldn't be reading this book now. The fact is that 90% of the existing medical information on gout is what mystifies gout and makes it look so complicated and incurable. It is only when you are still suffering from the disease they can keep on earning profits from selling painkillers to you.

If you want to be free from gout, you must first demystify gout. The first step is to unlearn what you have learned. Once you have gotten rid of the old perspective, open your mind to accept the new one that I'm going to share in the coming chapters.

Chapter 2

Gout Is Curable

Conventional medicine does not have the technology to get rid of the deposited urate crystals. Medicine can only use drugs to suppress the formation of new urate crystals and manage the pain. Doctors are taught that gout is incurable, and the doctors pass the same message to their patients as well. It's very sad and depressing to be told by a doctor that you have an incurable disease and have to depend on medications for the rest of your life.

The truth is that gout is not just a painful problem in your foot. It is actually a warning sign that your body is suffering from metabolic disorders that affect many aspect of your life. After interviewing hundreds of gout patients, I discovered that they actually share many other common health complications on top of the painful swollen joints. I've arranged these symptoms in chronological order and summarized them into the nine stages of gout.

Nine Stages of Gout

(Which stage are you at?)

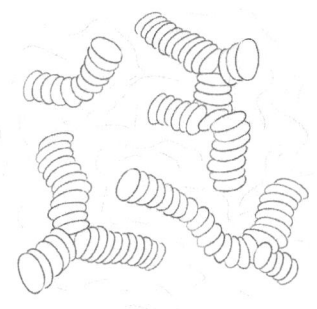

Figure 2.1 Red blood cells stack together

Stage 1: Your blood is thick and dark because of the high uric acid concentration.

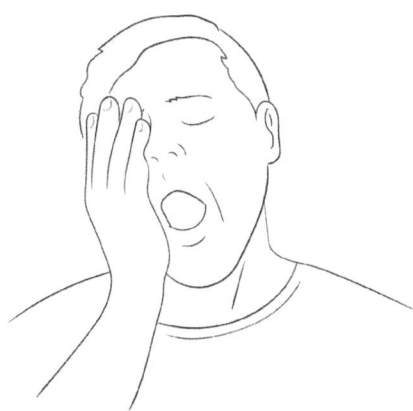

Figure 2.2 Sleepiness

Stage 2: You frequently feel tired and sleepy because of the slow-flowing blood.

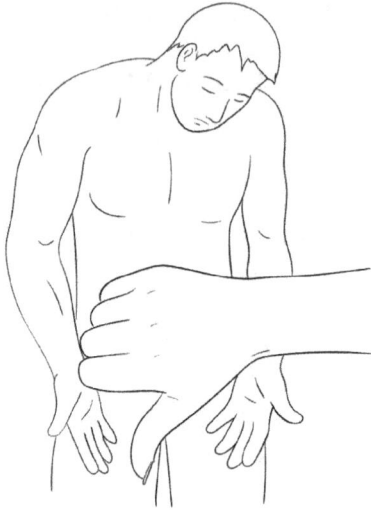

Figure 2.3 Low sex drive

Stage 3: There is significant drop in the level of your sexual desire and performance.

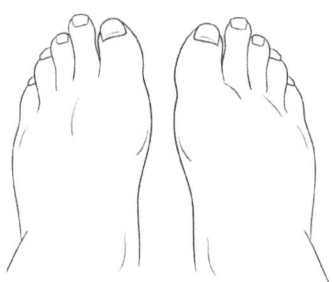

Figure 2.4 Swollen foot

Stage 4: Gout begins to attack your lower joints, especially the big toe, which causes intense pain and swelling.

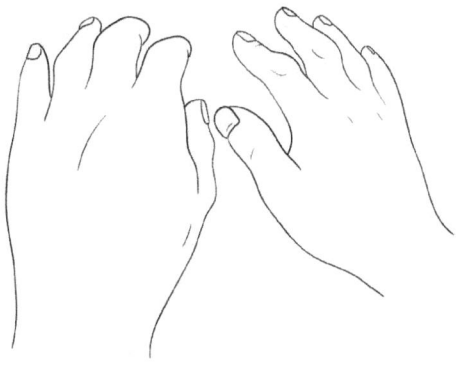

Figure 2.5 Swollen hand

Stage 5: The gout attacks start to "climb up" to the upper joints, such as your hands and elbows.

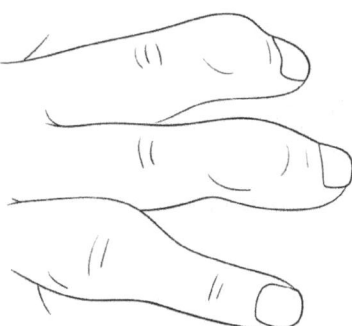

Figure 2.6 Unbendable fingers

Stage 6: Urate crystals cause permanent physical damages to the cartilage of smaller joints, such as your fingers, which makes them unbendable.

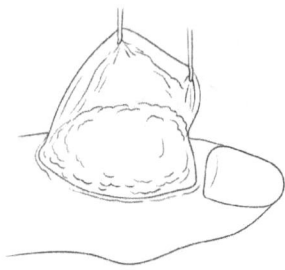

Figure 2.7 Tophi deposit in big toe

Stage 7: Tophi start forming near the skin surface. Most of the time, this begins near the ear lobes.

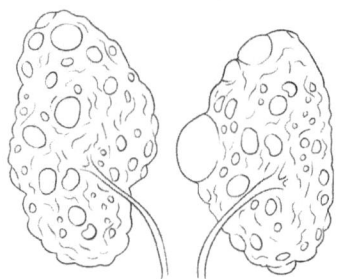

Figure 2.8 Damaged kidneys

Stage 8: Kidney function degenerates and kidney stones form. If left untreated, this will eventually lead to kidney failure.

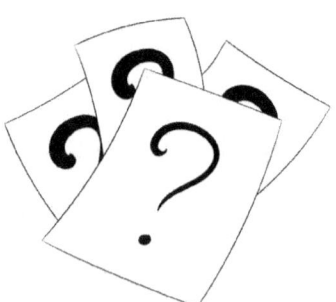

Figure 2.9 You guess

Final stage. (?)

If gout is predictable, there must be a pattern or root that can be tracked down. This means gout is indeed curable!

Gout Is Not a Complicated Problem

Treating gout is very simple, only if you understand the root of it. And there is only one cause of gout, only one: uric acid. Pain in the joints or muscles suffered by gout patients is caused by the crystallization of uric acid that forms inside the synovial fluid in the joints. These tiny needle-like crystals (monosodium urate) scratch the surface of hyaline cartilage and trigger a series of autoimmune reactions and pains commonly known as a gout attack.

High levels of uric acid in your body are a direct result of what you have put into your mouth through the years. We are surrounded by acidic food everywhere. High-protein, high-carbohydrate processed foods and carbonated drinks are all acidic.

Not only the food you eat but also your lifestyle can cause your body to produce more acids. Those who are living an "acidic lifestyle" are those who lack sleep, overwork, and are always under stress. If you fit into any of these criteria, go for a blood test now! Chances are that the uric acid reading of your blood is either on the high side or already way above the healthy range.

You might have heard people say that gout is not merely caused by hyperuricemia; it could also be caused by old age, hormonal changes, and genetic inheritance.

Old age? The youngest gout sufferer I know is only 19 years old. More than 50% of the gout patients that call my office to seek help are in their 20s or 30s. Most of the time, it is the wives of these young gout victims who have called for help because she feels sad to see her husband going through the torturing pain. It is just too young for a healthy man to have a notorious disease like gout that robs the happiness of the family.

Hormonal changes? More than 90% of gout patients are adult males in their mid-30s and older. Isn't that is a bit too early for them to go through hormonal changes? By the way, men do actually to go through menopause, I mean male menopause. As far as I know, a man goes through significant hormone change only when he is sexually aroused. Thus the theory suggesting gout is caused by hormone imbalance is rather absurd.

Genetic inheritance? This popular explanation is given by the medical professionals when they cannot explain why a father and son are suffering the same disease. To date, there is still little research that shows scientists have found the gene related to the regulation of uric acid levels. Many hundreds of years ago, gout occurred only among the small genetic pool of rich people. If the genetic inheritance theory of gout is true, why are there are so many people suffering from gout nowadays? Don't tell me the rich and famous in those days had fathered so many babies that they eventually grew to become the gout-prone generation we see now.

Ironically, many of the gout patients now are of lower income or poor groups who find it hard to continuously pay for the gout medication that is getting more and more expensive.

I have come across so many cases in which almost all the adult males in a family suffer from gout. That has made me wonder what is the missing link. It was after many conversations with the gout patients that I've finally found the answer that explains why gout shows the trend of inheritance.

If we forget about the aspect of DNA or genetics, gout is actually a hereditary disease. But it is not genetically related. I call that a "diet lifestyle heredity." Since the day a baby boy is born, chances are very high that he will copy the diet habits of his parents. He will favor what his father favors. If the father loves high-purine food—such as red meat (think weekend family BBQs), peas, and beans—for sure the loving dad will share the delicious food with his beloved son. And that is when the seed of gout is planted. This leads us back to the one and only root of gout: high levels of uric acid.

There is only one cause of gout, only one: uric acid.

Allopurinol Does Not Flush Away Uric Acid

You might complain that the gout pain still attacks even though you have totally cut off high-purine food, which is the raw material of uric acid production in the body. The uric acid level in your blood doesn't seem to show any significant reduction even though you have been continuously taking allopurinol or other similar medicines.

Allopurinol is a xanthine oxidase inhibitor, which suppresses the degradation of purine into uric acid. It is like blocking your car exhaust pipe with a banana. Xanthine oxidase helps rid the human body of the excessive purine by breaking it down into uric acid for disposal through the kidneys. But our smart scientists have invented something call allopurinol to interrupt that process.

Where Are Those Undisposed Purines Stored in the Body Then?

Purine is broken down in the liver. If there is too much deposited purine left in the liver, it adds to the burden of the organ and eventually leads to liver failure. In some cases, the purines reenter the bloodstream and seek alternative ways out, which is through the skin. That explains why some people experience skin problems after they consume allopurinol.

Allopurinol can prevent the uric acid in your body from increasing, but it cannot get rid of the uric acid that has already accumulated all over your body over the years, especially when it has crystallized in the joints. You will continue to suffer from gout attacks in the future if you don't take the initiative to neutralize and flush out hidden uric acid in you body. Your gout problem is cured only after you have successfully flushed away the excess uric acid from your body. Remember, gout is curable.

Chapter 3

Cellular Biology

To demystify gout, we must look at the problem beyond the painful big toe. We have to see through it by understanding the problem from inside out, which is at the cellular level. That's why I have to explain some basic cellular biology here to help you understand how ionized alkaline water actually works in flushing the unwanted uric acid from your body.

The human body always works to maintain a blood pH of 7.4, which is mildly alkaline. When there are too many acidic chemicals in the blood as a result of an acidic diet or emotional stress, the body triggers a series of homeostatic reactions to raise the blood pH to its optimum level. One mechanism used by the blood is to move the excess acidic compounds, such as uric acid, out of the bloodstream.

Interstitial Fluid

Interstitial fluid (or tissue fluid) is a solution that bathes and surrounds the cells of multicellular animals. It is the main component of the extracellular fluid, which also includes plasma and transcellular fluid. The interstitial fluid is found in the interstitial spaces, also known as the tissue spaces.

The direct deposit site of uric acids is the interstitial fluid between the capillaries and cells, as shown in **Figure 3.1**. Initially, interstitial fluid is just like a temporary storage site for any excess acids until the blood pH is back to normal and can slowly transport those uric acids to the kidneys for removal through urine. But if you continuously eat acidic food (not only high-purine food) and drink acidic drinks (high sugar and carbonated), there is no chance for your body to get rid of those "refugee" acids in the interstitial fluid.

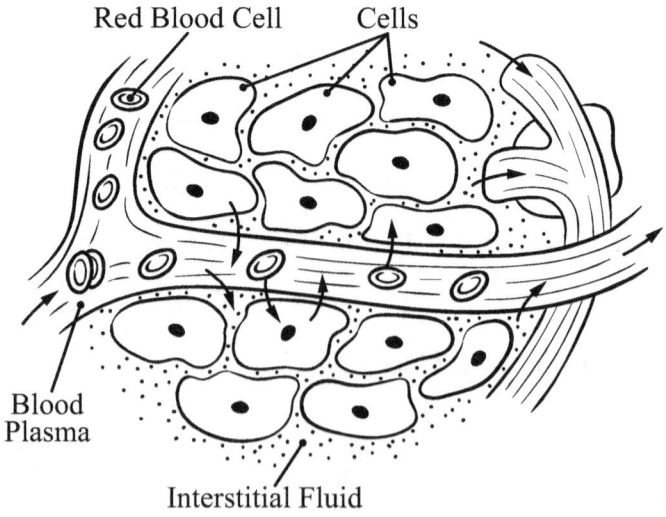

Figure 3.1 Deposit site of uric acids

When the acid content of interstitial fluid climbs higher, it forces some acid to seep further and deeper until it reaches the synovial fluid in the joints. Eventually, when the concentration of uric acid in the joint reaches the saturation point, it crystallizes and forms needle-like monosodium urate crystals.

Seed Crystal

A seed crystal is a small piece of crystal material from which a larger crystal of the same material typically can be grown. In solution, soluble molecules are free to move about in a random flow. This random flow may allow two or more molecular compounds to interact and form the basis for a crystal network. The entrance of a seed crystal into solution accelerates the crystallization process by eliminating the need for random molecular interaction. With a target crystal to act upon, the molecular interactions occur much more easily than by relying on a random flow. Seeding is therefore said to decrease the amount of time needed for the crystallization process.

Given the right temperature and concentration, a tiny seed crystal of uric acid can form in less than a second and then quickly grow to a needle-like urate crystal structure in minutes. As soon as our natural immune system detects these solid crystals, it considers them foreign pathogens, and a series of immune defenses triggers in no time. Inflammation, a burning sensation, and extreme pain soon follow. This autoimmune reaction feels exactly the same as being stung by a poisonous bee.

Crystallization happens much more easily at lower temperatures. This explains why the onset of most gout attacks occurs at night, especially during winter. Even while you are sleeping soundly, it can wake you suddenly.

You should now have a clearer picture of how uric acid travels into the joints and forms urate crystals that later trigger a gout attack. Let's get back to the main question of this chapter …

Why Do Some People Suffer from Gout Attacks Even Though Their Blood Uric Acid Reading Is Low?

To answer this question, I have come up with the Black Box theory of gout that will help simplify the crystallization process and make it easier to understand (**Figure 3.2**).

The Gout Black Box Reaction

The journey of uric acids from the blood plasma into the synovial fluid in the joints is not a direct process. The rate at which uric acids become urate crystals in the joints and how fast the immune system kick-starts the inflammation reactions varies from one patient to another. Let's assume the complicated processes between uric acids in the blood and the onset of a gout attack happens as shown by the gout black box reaction.

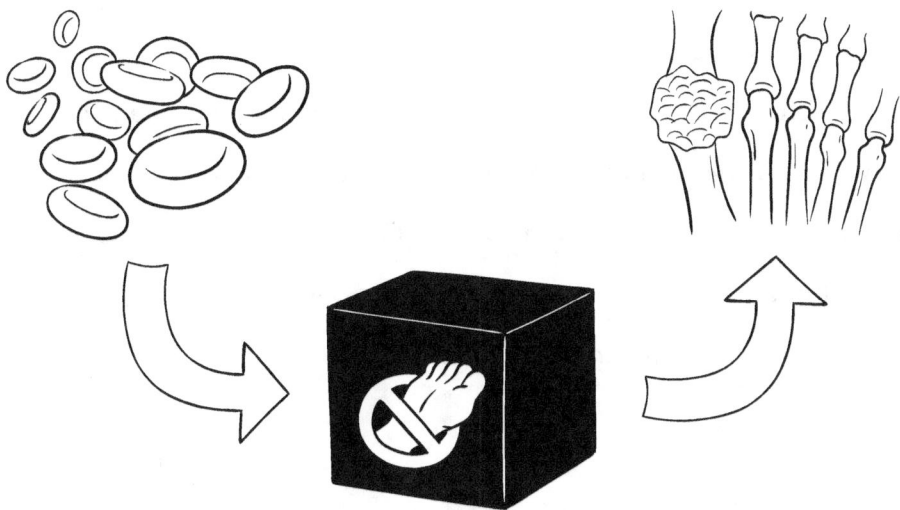

Figure 3.2 The Gout Black Box Reaction

Some people's gout black box is very fast and effective in transforming uric acids into urate crystals; these are the gout patients who always have a healthy level of uric acid reading in their blood test reports. Since blood tests can never indicate the existence of urate crystals in the joints, the only way to confirm it is through arthroscopic surgery or synovial fluid analysis.

On the other hand, some patients have a slower gout black box, which is not good at channeling those excess uric acids out of the blood stream to the joint. Those uric acids either stay in the blood or stick in the interstitial fluid and eventually develop into tophi, which pop out from the surface of the skin. These people have constant high blood uric acid readings but seldom or never suffer from gout attacks.

Another group of gout patients consists of those who have high uric acid readings and frequently suffer from gout attacks. Their gout black box is working neither too fast nor too slow. I wouldn't say it is normal because a normal, healthy person never needs this gout black box at all.

The Gout Black Box theory is a very important paradigm shift toward a true gout cure. Read on to have a better understanding of this notorious disease. By the time you've finished reading this book, you should have a very clear understanding of gout, and you will absolutely know what you should do to cure it once and for all.

Chapter 4

Acidosis and Thick Blood

One of the common symptoms felt by those suffering from hyperuricemia or gout is that they feel tired or sluggish most of the time. Most gout patients find it hard to have good quality sleep and often wake up with a blurry mind that needs at least half an hour to clear up.

What Causes This?

If you look at their freshly drawn blood, you will notice almost all of these patients have thick blood, dark in color with high viscosity. If you observe the blood under darkfield microscopy, you will notice the red blood cells are stacking up in clusters.

With thick blood, the red blood cells cannot carry as much oxygen as is possible; they cannot bring fresh oxygen to the muscles, to the lungs, or any other parts of the body, especially the brain. We need a fast and sufficient supply of oxygen to the brain so we can think clearly and concisely.

Thick blood is a condition that creeps up on us over a long period. It can slowly disturb our quality of life if the situation is ignored.

What Are the Consequences?

A person having thick blood can get an array of seemingly unrelated symptoms that will send the doctors scratching their heads.

Here are some of those symptoms:

• **Skin disorders—such as red patches, itchiness, acne, and dryness and flaking—sometimes misdiagnosed as eczema or dermatitis:** This thick blood is not efficient in carrying toxins to the liver or kidneys for disposal. This has forced the body to go for the next available eliminative organ: the skin. Our skin is the largest organ, in terms of surface area, and has millions of pores or openings. Our body is constantly eliminating excess water, toxins, and heat via those pores on the skin. When the kidneys and liver fail to take the load off the laboring red blood cells, they have no choice but to dump their load on the next available channel, which is the skin. This is why the skin gets dry, itchy, flaking, red, or swollen—to help cleanse the blood so it can continue doing its work.

• **Migraines or headaches:** The brain does not receive enough oxygen from the blood when it is submerged in an environment full of toxic waste that cannot be transported out for disposal. Frequently a headache for no obvious reason is the signal that your brain is shouting for help. As long as the blood is not cleaned up, you will always have headaches that come and go. When your blood cannot carry sufficient oxygen and nutrients to the brain cells, they become tired, and the ability to spark signals drops. The result is lapses of memory, forgetfulness, and lack of concentration, which will eventually affect the quality of your daily life.

- **Fever or high body temperature that comes and goes:** A fever is one of the body's immune responses that attempts to neutralize a bacterial or viral infection. However, if your blood is too thick, certain toxic wastes become concentrated and mimic foreign substances. When the immune "police" spot these toxins, they raise the temperature a degree or so as an attempt to burn out these waste toxins. The typical medical doctor assumes that you have a virus or a bacterial infection and prescribes a universal weapon for you: antibiotics. This kind of fever shows up from time to time with no periodic cycle evident. After about two or three trips to the doctor, the doctor may draw some blood from you to see what monsters are hiding inside your body. Guess what he will find out next.

- **High white blood cell count:** If your lab reports come back with a high white blood cell count—even after antibiotics—consider the possibility that it is an autoimmune reaction where the body tries to kill off those toxins. When that happens, there is an elevated or higher white blood cell count, which the doctors verify as bacteria or a virus still active and in your body. There have been some cases where the white blood count was so high that the condition was diagnosed as preleukemic.

- **Various forms of unknown allergic reactions:** A high concentration of toxic compounds in the body can force the immune system into a major reaction. After several years, it goes haywire, becoming weak and suppressed or overly sensitive. As the immune system begins to turn upside down, you suddenly become allergic to something in your environment. Allergies are signals that your immune system is wearing down and will eventually leave you open to all kinds of problems later, such as more frequent flu or other deadly forms of bacteria and viruses. Your main line of defense has been stripped of its protective powers and is leaving you wide open to all these other risks.

After knowing all the consequences of having a thick blood, the next question is …

What Causes the Blood to Become Thick?

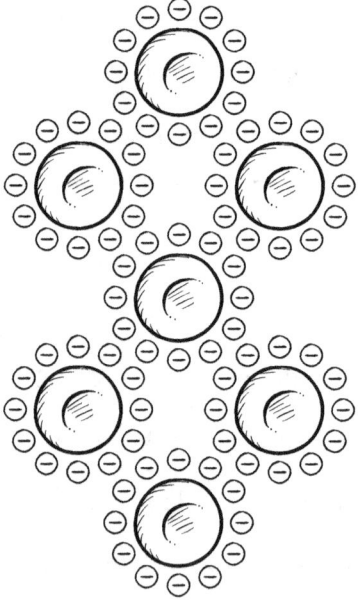

Figure 4.1 High zeta potential

Every cell in the body has an electrical potential, especially on the surface of its membrane. It is this electrical energy that differentiates life from death. The electrical potential, also known as zeta potential, ranges from 70 to 90 millivolts in a healthy human cell.

Zeta potential is a measure of the electrical force that exists between atoms, molecules, particles, and cells in a fluid. Zeta potential's strength determines the amount of material (nutrients or wastes) that fluids, such as blood and lymph, can

carry. Increasing the electrical force in the solution allows the fluid to dissolve and hold more material. In this way, more nutrients can be carried throughout your body and accumulated deposits of waste can be removed.

A high zeta potential is the ability of a molecule to hold an electrical charge. Zeta potential is the force that maintains the discreteness of each cell in our body. As we age or become ill, our zeta potential drops, along with our energy. If you find it difficult to get out of bed, exercise, or maintain self-motivation, don't blame it on your psychological state. It could be due to the low zeta potential at the cell level.

Healthy red blood cells are fully charged with negative ions on the membrane surface. Under normal conditions, it is hard for two or more red blood cells to get near each other because negative charges repel each other. In the case of blood, more negative ions means higher zeta potential.

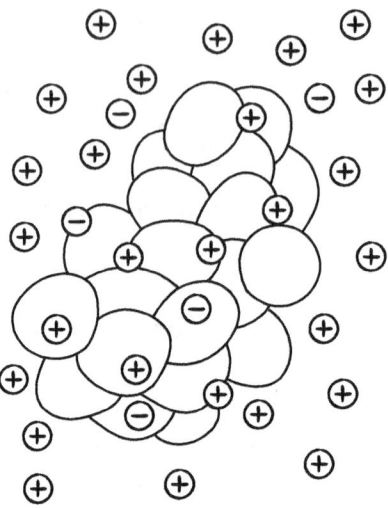

Figure 4.2 Low Zeta Potential

If there is too much uric acid in the blood, a lot of positively charged hydrogen ions float around in the blood plasma. These positively charged ions neutralize the negative charges on the red blood cells. Eventually, this leads to a drop of zeta potential in the blood. When the zeta potential is too low, blood begins to coagulate. This condition is known as intravascular coagulation. Blood becomes a sludge, which I call "thick blood," that is increasingly difficult for the heart to pump, and it becomes ineffective performing the normal blood functions.

Gout Is Just the Beginning

Gout is just one of the ways your body calls for help; it is one of the earliest warning signs that your body is heading toward acidosis. Just like a house full of dirty rubbish, pests (mice and cockroaches) will keep coming in no matter how hard you try to eliminate them. It is a never-ending process. My advice: stop wasting time and money trying to kill those nasty pests. Focus on cleaning house instead and throwing away all the rubbish. When it is clean and tidy, mice and cockroaches and other pests gradually go away because that is no longer the environment they seek. Cleaning house might appear harder than setting traps for mice and bugs, but which one do you prefer? Setting up traps every day or cleaning house once and for all?

The same concept applies to your body. There is no instant cure for anything. You didn't get gout today or yesterday; your gouty enemy began forming many years back and started to attack only recently. So, don't expect there to be an instant cure for a disease 10 years in the making. Those meds you take are just a smoke screen that masks your pain and symptoms, which makes you think that the illness is cured. Sadly, the effectiveness of the meds is just temporary. Soon you will have another round of gout attacks.

Pharmaceutical drugs and medicines cannot cure modern illnesses, and they gradually pollute your body's internal environment, eventually leading to other diseases. By now, you should know why you still suffer from gout symptoms no matter how much colchicine, allopurinol, and painkiller you take.

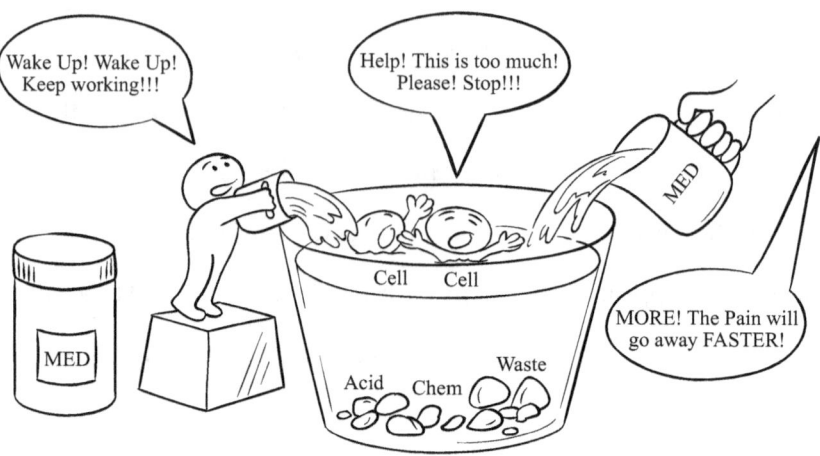

Figure 4.3 Pharmaceutical drugs pollution

Most of us know the benefits of detoxification, but knowing without practicing is as good as nothing. It requires strong personal strength and self-discipline to achieve it. You are what you eat and drink. Your lifestyle determines the internal living condition for your body's cells. If you always consume acidic food and drinks, the cells in your body will be surrounded by the same thing too.

Gout is a habitual disease. It sprouted from some of your habits, especially your daily diet.

I know it is hard to change a habit, so take it one step at a time. I believe that with a clear understanding on the origin of gout, you'll have a better understanding of how to balance your diet. Remember to always keep the balance. Great food is one of the pleasures of life, so enjoy it. But always know the limits. A simple principle I practice to stay healthy at all time is this: If yesterday's diet was high in acidic protein and meat, then today must be an alkaline-vegetarian type of day to balance it. Try it. Don't forget the most important element of detoxification. Drink plenty of good water, preferably ionized alkaline water, frequently during the day.

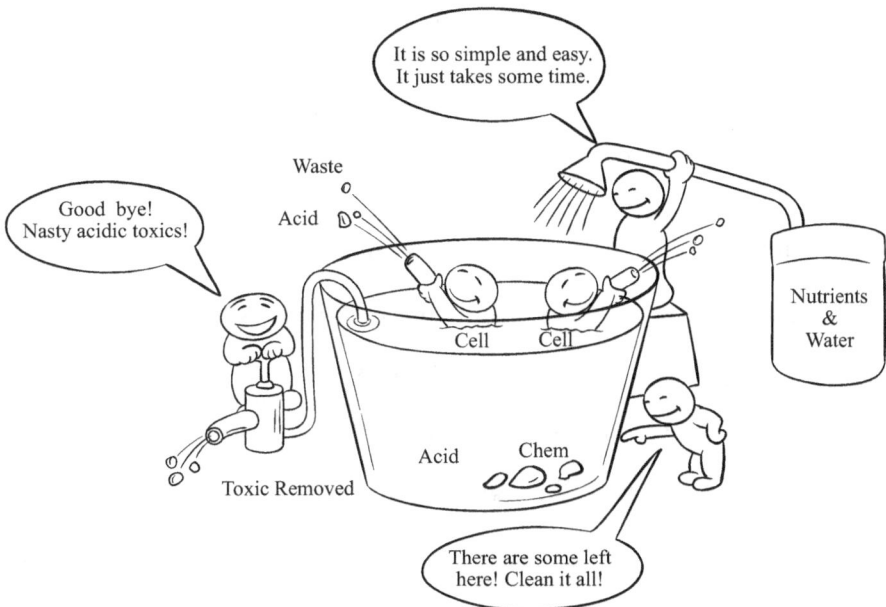

Figure 4.4 Nutrients & water detoxification

How Much Water Should You Drink a Day?

Forget about the "eight glasses of water a day" saying. That can be very confusing and misleading. The glasses in your kitchen are probably a different size from those in your neighbor's cabinet. So, how about two liters a day? What about three?

How much water to drink a day differs from person to person and depends on one's daily activities. A rule of thumb is to drink at least 5% of your body weight (in metric units). Take me as an example: My weight is around 70 kilograms. I drink at least three and a half liters of ionized alkaline water in a day.

The 5% Rule

Take in at least 5% of your body weight (in metric units) of ionized alkaline water daily.

I know for some of you, drinking three and a half liters of water in a day might sound ridiculous, if not crazy. And I'm very sure at least 90% of you reading this are heavier than I am, which means you might need to drink up to five liters of water per day, according to the 5% rule. Your doctor is going to tell you, "This guy is a nut job."

Tell me, who is the bigger nut: someone who gives you advice and meds proven not to cure disease or me? Big Pharma would have been out of business a long time ago if their meds cured anything. You wouldn't be reading this e-book if those prescriptions worked.

Here is the logic of my 5% rule. Trace back the history of human evolution billions of years, and all living things on earth originated from a single cell formed in the sea of water. The human body is a very complex combination of one hundred trillion (100,000,000,000,000) living cells. These cells exist in a sea of interstitial body fluids just like an enclosed sea where they get their food supply. Blood capillaries act as the tiny rivers that supply the nutrients to this huge internal sea of cells.

Now imagine an aquarium with 100 fish inside. More fish means more waste will be produced. Guess how long it takes for the tank of clear water to turn dirty and murky. Less than three days. You have to either change the water or kiss the fish good-bye. So, you install a pump system to recycle and filter out the waste made by the fish. Then, once a week, you need to change the filter sponges and flush the line out so the pump system operates smoothly.

Now imagine one hundred trillion fish cramped in a relatively small tank. Our body has a built-in recycling system that pumps very hard to filter out those toxic wastes. But we cannot change out the filtering sponges in our body (kidneys) to scrub or rinse them. The only way to clean them is to flush our system with water and excrete urine. The same principle applies to another filtering organ: the skin.

Caution!

Watch out for water poisoning! Never gulp down more than one liter of water—especially pure water, such as reversed osmosis water and distilled water—within minutes. Too much pure water will dilute the electrolytes in your body, which could result in seizures, brain damage, coma, or even death!

The best drinking water practice is a moderate amount with high frequency, such as 500 milliliters every hour or so. If you are not a water-drinking person, chances are high that your kidneys have grown lazy. So, allow some time for their muscles to gradually remember this flushing job. If you seldom run or exercise and then, out of the blue, run a 10K race, guess how you will feel the next day. I doubt if you would be able get out of bed. You see, those muscles had grown lazy too. Get it?

If 5% of your weight is a bit too much for you, you can cut it down to 3% for a start. What is important is that you have to work out your number so that you have something to aim for, achieve, and then stick to.

Warning!

If you have a weak kidney or any other kidney illness.
DO NOT practice the 5% rule.

Chapter 5

Gout and Kidney Stones

At least half of all gout patients will have a kidney stone (ureterolithiasis) problem if their hyperuricemia goes untreated for years. Some people say the weakened kidneys' inability to filter out excess uric acid causes the elevation of uric acid in the blood. If so, then what causes one's kidneys to fail to do their job? Before I can answer that question, I must help you recall what is taught about the kidneys in high school biology classes.

Know Your Kidneys

As one of the vital organs of the human body, the kidneys perform several essential tasks, including the excretion of waste products, the maintenance of homeostatic balance in the body, and the release of important hormones. To achieve this, human kidneys have a highly developed, superbly refined anatomy and physiology.

The kidneys are bean-shaped organs, each about the size of a fist (10 centimeters long and 6.5 centimeters wide). Each is identical in structure and function. They are located near the middle of the back, just below the rib cage, one on each side of the spine. The kidneys are sophisticated reprocessing machines. In healthy adults, about 180 liters of fluid is filtered into the kidney tubules each day. Nearly all this fluid and the electrolytes contained in it are reabsorbed by the kidney; only about 2% is excreted as urine. The wastes and extra water become urine, which flows to the bladder through tubes called ureters. The bladder stores urine until releasing it through urination. (See **Figure 5.1.**)

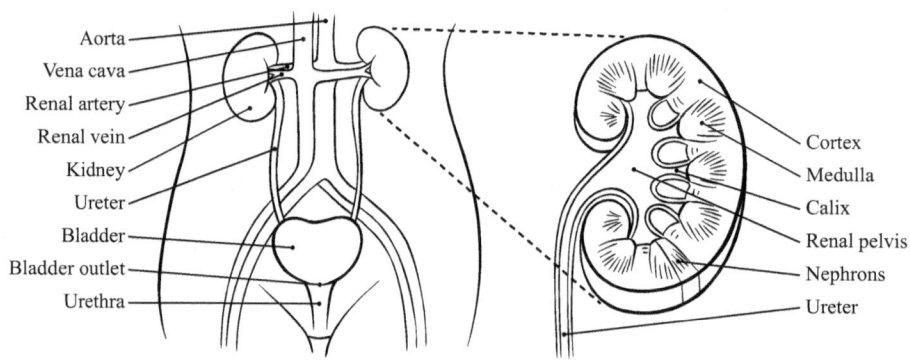

Figure 5.1 The human urinary system

Wastes in the blood come from the normal breakdown of active tissues, such as muscles, and from food. The body uses food for energy and self-repairs. After the body has taken what it needs from food, wastes are sent to the blood. If the kidneys do not remove them, these wastes build up in the blood and damage the body.

Each kidney comprises an outer cortex and an inner medulla. The kidney is supplied with oxygenated blood via the renal artery and drained of deoxygenated blood by the renal vein. In addition, urine produced by the kidney as part of its excretory function drains out via narrow tubules and the ureter to the bladder. (See **Figure 5.2**.)

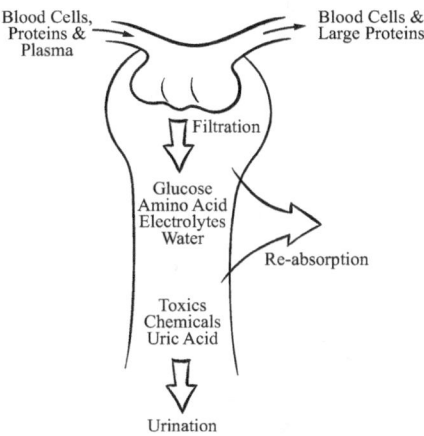

Figure 5.2 The kindeys' excretory process

The actual removal of wastes occurs in tiny units inside the kidneys called nephrons. Each kidney has about a million nephrons. In the nephron, a glomerulus—which is a tiny blood vessel, or capillary—intertwines with a tiny urine-collecting tube called a tubule. The glomerulus acts as a filtering unit, or sieve, and keeps normal proteins and cells in the bloodstream, allowing extra fluid and wastes to pass through. A complicated chemical exchange takes place as waste materials and water leave the blood and enter the urinary system.

At first, the tubules receive a combination of waste materials and chemicals the body can still use. The kidneys measure out sodium, phosphorus, and potassium and release them back to the blood to return to the body. In this way, the kidneys regulate the body's level of these and other substances. The right balance is necessary for life.

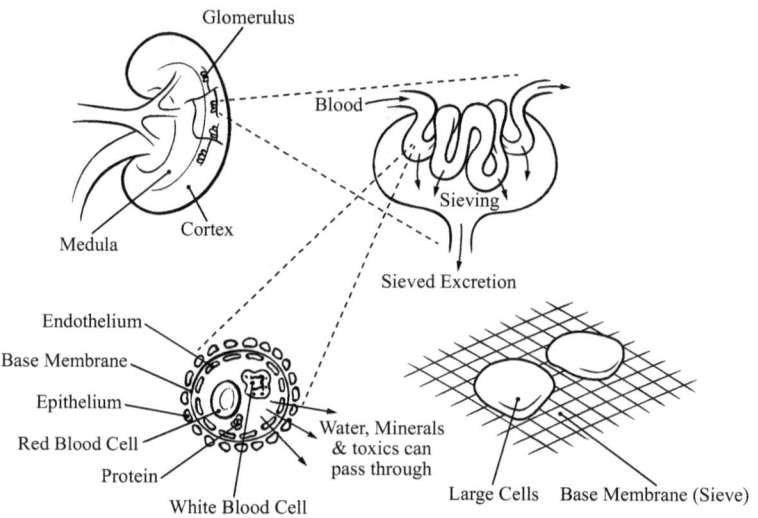

Figure 5.3 The kidneys' regulatory process

It is estimated that the total filtration capacity of both kidneys within one minute for a healthy person is between 100 ~ 150 milliliters (125 milliliters). This value is known as the Glomerular Filtration rate. As long as there is blood flowing through the glomerulus, the filtration process will happens automatically.

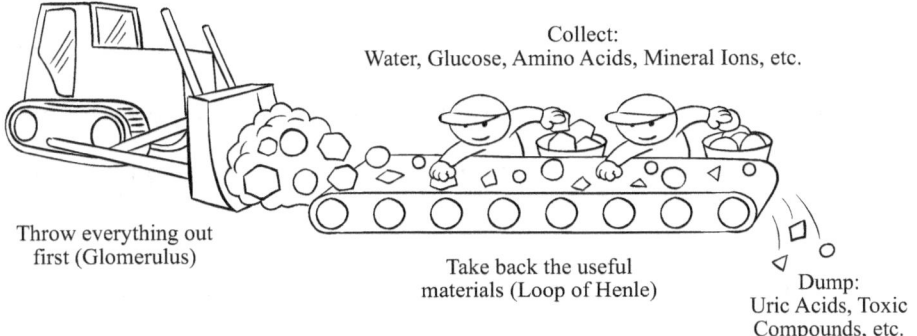

Collect:
Water, Glucose, Amino Acids, Mineral Ions, etc.

Throw everything out
first (Glomerulus)

Take back the useful
materials (Loop of Henle)

Dump:
Uric Acids, Toxic
Compounds, etc.

Figure 5.4 The kidneys' filtration process

Up to 60% of the human body is water. The brain is comprised of 70% water, and the lungs are nearly 90% water. Lean muscle tissue contains about 75% water by weight, as does the brain; body fat contains 10% water, and bone has 22% water. About 85% of our blood is water, which helps digest our food, transport waste, and control body temperature. Each day humans must replace at least two and half liters of water, some through drinking and the rest taken by the body from the foods eaten.

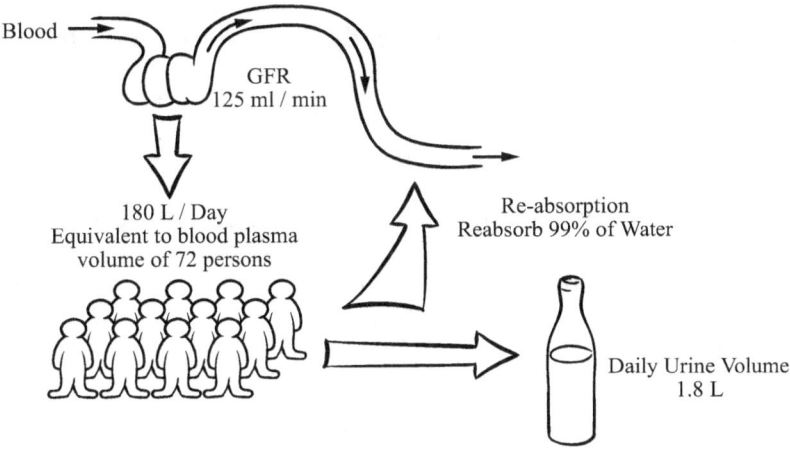

Blood

GFR
125 ml / min

180 L / Day
Equivalent to blood plasma
volume of 72 persons

Re-absorption
Reabsorb 99% of Water

Daily Urine Volume
1.8 L

Figure 5.5 The reabsorption mechanism

Within 24 hours, there will be 144 ~ 216 liters (average, 180 liters) being filtered through those 2 millions tiny glomeruli in the kidneys (**Figure 5.5**). Imagine if there were no reabsorption mechanism, we would have to either consume 180 liters of water every day or become dried up within hours!

Luckily, 99% of the water is reabsorbed back to the blood as soon as it comes out from the glomerulus. The other 1% of water is used to flush out wastes and toxics from the kidney.

What Will Happen if a Person Does Not Drink Enough Water?

About 85% of our blood is made of water. When there is not enough water in the blood, our body sends out signals to the kidney to reabsorb more water back into the blood to compensate for this water deficit. This results in much lower water content in the urine produced. In another words, urine becomes very thick or saturated. If you are hyperuricemic, try collecting your urine in a transparent plastic cup and leave it somewhere safe overnight. Look at it the next day, paying close attention to the bottom of the cup. You will notice some fine tiny sediment formed there. If you do not pass urine as often and as much as you should, there will be not enough water to flush away the toxic wastes in the kidney tubules. Accumulation of this uric acid (dried) is how crystallization of kidney stones begins.

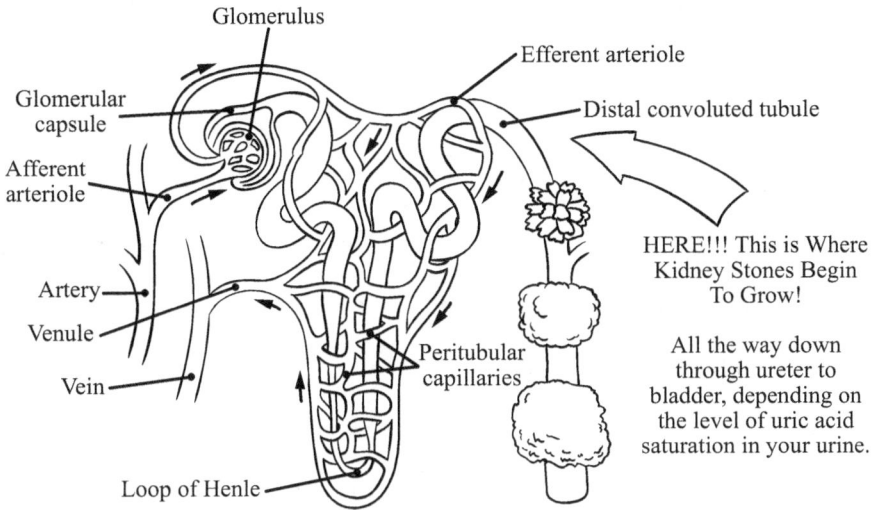

Figure 5.6 The development of kidney stones

About 90% of kidney stone patients do not have the habit of drinking water frequently. (I mean plain drinking water or mineral water). The ironic part is that they often do not realize that their body is crying for more water. They always claim that they drink plenty of water during the day. Well, the water is in fact liquids: soft drinks, beer, tea, coffee, milk, juices, or any other drinkable liquids.

This is a big "no-no." Those drinks will only make you thirst more for water. Go grab a bottle of beer now and finish it, and I guarantee that you will feel thirstier within 30 minutes. All right, you might say, alcohol is commonly known to be dehydrating. Then trying drinking a bottle of cola or any sweet syrup juice, and you will get the same result.

All these modern drinks are full of excess ingredients, especially sugar or artificial sweeteners and colorings. Consuming these drinks makes your blood become thicker or hypertonic, which will absorb water out from the interstitial fluids or body cells. Gradually, your body cells become dryer and dryer.

Under such conditions, the kidneys have to reduce the excretion of water into the urine to keep enough water to maintain the blood concentration. This results in thick and highly saturated urine that flows slowly through the ureter. Hypermaturation is the perfect condition for crystallization to happen. If it continues for a certain period of time, the tiny crystal grows bigger until it blocks the passage of the urine. This blockage causes the pressure to build up in the kidney, so now the kidney is forced to squeeze the urethral muscle to force the urine trough the small passage. This is when the patient starts to feel some pain.

Warning!

If you feel some odd pain at the lower part of you back, slightly above your hips, go in for a blood test to check your uric acid level.

If the result of a blood test to check your uric acid level is way above healthy range, chances are high that there are already some crystal stones (maybe still too tiny to be seen through an X-ray) in your kidneys. Take action before it is too late because you will not like the way the doctors break those stones. Try to imagine someone sliding a long fine tubing through your private part, and then twisting and poking with it to break down or remove those stubborn stones. Don't you think cultivating a good water drinking habit is a much better option?

The following chapters will introduce to you different types of drinking water available in the market. The last chapter of this book will show the right type of water and how to begin drinking it to neutralize the accumulated uric acid effectively.

Chapter 6

Pure Water

Pure water is the cleanest water on earth; it does not contain any pollutants or minerals. It is pure H2O only. There are two methods to produce pure water: distillation and reverse osmosis.

Distillation: Distilled Water

Do you still remember the experiment as shown in **Figure 6.1**? It is one of the earliest experiments that we learned in science class. Many centuries ago, the distillation process was utilized to produce strong liquors, such as vodka and whisky.

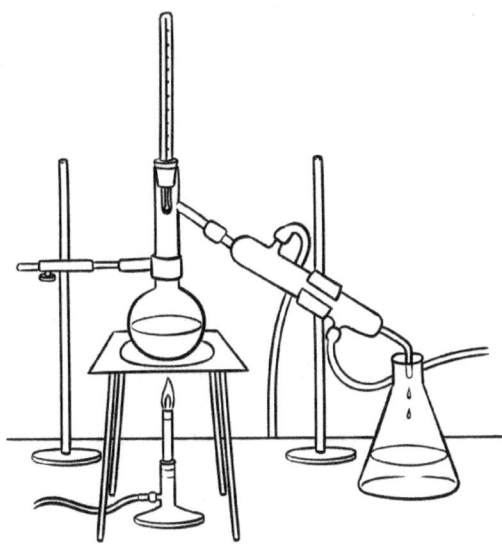

Figure 6.1 Apparatus for distilling water

After the advent of modern science, distillation became widely used in labs to produce pure water for use in scientific experiments. Since the 1980s, distilled water has become one of the most popular drinking waters for the general public. This is because some "experts" claim that drinking the purest water cleanses the body and promotes health.

This notion was first made popular when someone invented the office drinking water machine, which has hot and cold taps dispensing the distilled water from a huge five-gallon blue bottle (**Figure 6.2**).

Not long after that, some entrepreneurs observed big potential in the household market, so they invented some cute little distillation machine called the RainMaker, as shown in **Figure 6.3**.

The RainMaker can produce distilled drinking water without any water supply. The salespeople who promote these "stills" claim this machine can make water from the air. Amazing? Not really.

Actually, the operating concept behind this cute little RainMaker is quite simple: it condenses the moisture in the air so that it drops into a glass container. This machine is just a tiny refrigerator with some thin metal blades that are cooled to a very low temperature.

When the tiny, lightweight water molecules in the air hit a cold blade, they lose their kinetic energy and bond to form heavier water drops. They flow to a collecting tray and come out via the tiny output tap, drop by drop. Depending on the amount of moisture in the air where you live, it could take you at least 10 minutes to get a glass of drinking water using this machine.

Actually, you can produce fresh distilled water anytime at home. Do you remember how a can of ice-cold cola or beer turns wet and slippery as soon as you take it out of the fridge? That condensation is distilled water. Do this enough times and you could have a glass of distilled water to drink.

That is a much cheaper method than the expensive RainMaker, which squeezes money out of thin air for the salesperson. It can cost up to USD $2,000 to buy a single minifridge that cannot store any food but is able to produce a few drops of pure water.

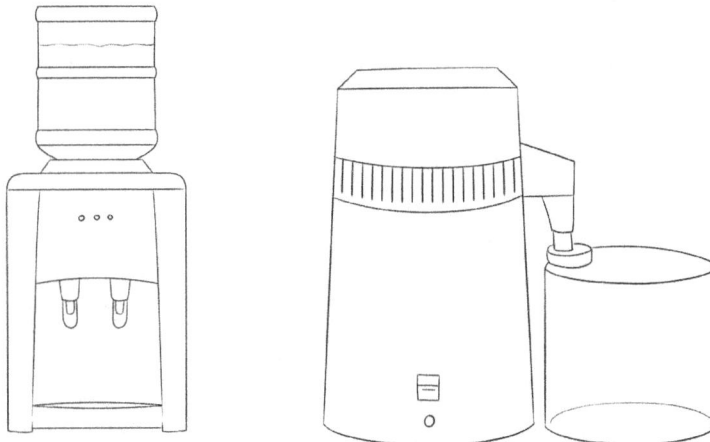

Figure 6.2 The ubiquitous blue water bottle

Figure 6.3 The cute little RainMaker

Reverse Osmosis: R. O. Water

Reverse osmosis is a relatively new technology for producing pure water. In this process, strong pressure is applied to one side of a filtering membrane that allows only water molecules to pass through. The water forced to cross through the membrane becomes pure water once it reaches the other side.

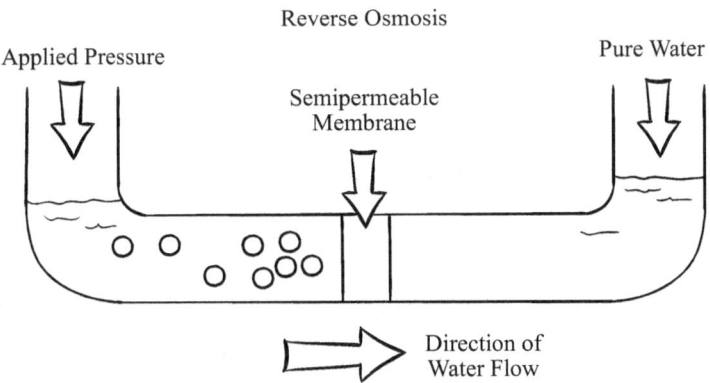

Figure 6.4 Reverse osmosis technology

Initially, reverse osmosis technology was used for industrial purposes in some small island countries. For example, Singapore uses it to process seawater into pure water, which is then mixed with water purchased from neighboring countries.

During the early 1990s, a few smaller-version R.O. machines were made available for household use. These were first promoted by some multilevel marketing (MLM) or direct selling companies and were sold at very high prices.

Some salespeople use various tricks to show how clean their R.O. water is and how dirty other drinking waters are. One popular trick is the use of a "water dirtiness" test device.

As soon as the salesperson enters your house, he will ask for a glass of your usual drinking water. He will then pour his R.O. water into an empty glass. After lining up the two glasses of water, he will take out his secret weapon, a small handheld total dissolved solids (TDS) test kit.

First, he will dip the TDS meter into his pure R.O. water; the reading on the LCD display will show "0." The salesperson explains that this measurement unit tests for how dirty your water is, and, obviously, the dirtiness of his R.O. water is zero!

Then he will dip the TDS meter into your current drinking water, and the number will show anything between "005" and "200." "Oh my! Look at this! Your water is not safe for drinking!" shouts the salesperson. Then his sales talk begins in earnest: blah, blah, blah … .

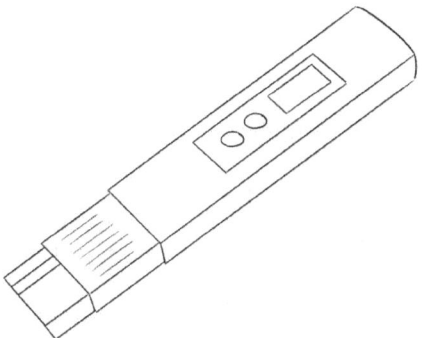

FIGURE 6.5 TDS meter

A TDS meter as shown in **Figure 6.5** is used to measure the quantity of minerals dissolved in water, but it is not a good measurement for how dirty your water is. Obviously, that trick is very misleading, and it instills fear in you so that you will be more open to his sales pitch.

Here is a way to undo that misleading trick. Wait until he has completed his demo and right after he tells you that a high TDS reading means your water is toxic or unhealthy, you go get a pinch of salt or milk powder from your kitchen and put it in his R.O. water. Ask him to test his R.O. water again. Voila! The reading should shoot above "200" or show "Err" which stands for error. Then you ask that salesperson, "Does this mean my salt or milk is super toxic?"

In some countries, distilled or R.O. water is sold in the form of bottled water. Usually, the government health department will make it compulsory for the bottles of all processed water, including distilled water and R.O. water, to use a white color cap. This is to differentiate those processed waters from natural mineral water, which uses blue or green color caps.

What Is the pH of Pure Water?

Theoretically, the pH of pure water is neutral, but when you test it with a pH tester, you will be surprised at the result. It is acidic. This surprises most professionals because they always think that pure water is neutral in pH because it contains no mineral that changes its pH.

Distilled water and R.O. water are acidic because they are too "empty." In nature, water is seldom found in its purest form because it has a unique feature (hydrogen bond), which makes it the universal solvent. This is why water is said to be fundamental to all living organisms.

Water from the river, sea, well, or even the rain, contains all sorts of dissolved minerals. But when water is processed through distillation or reverse osmosis, it becomes empty. Water will try to pull something in to fill this emptiness. The very first element it will absorb is carbon dioxide (CO_2) from the air.

When carbon dioxide is dissolved in water, it becomes carbonic acid, which gives the mild acidity found in pure water. Carbon dioxide and water molecules both have a similar three-atom structure; this creates a strong affinity between CO_2 and H_2O. This is why carbon dioxide gas is pumped into soft drinks to give them the fizzy sensation.

Then How Can We Get Really Pure Water?

Heat it up to slightly below the boiling point. This chases away all the dissolved carbon dioxide and gives you the purest pure water possible; but it is too hot to drink.

What Is the Benefit of Drinking Pure Water for Gout Patients?

Pure water does not contain any alkaline minerals that can help neutralize the acidic wastes that cause hyperuricemia. On the contrary, long-term drinking of pure water will dilute the essential electrolytes or minerals, which are important for the biochemical and metabolic processes in your body.

It makes perfect sense: you drink pure water without minerals, and when you go to the toilet, you eliminate urine that contains minerals. Where did the minerals in the urine come from? From your body! Keep drinking pure water for a few months or so, and eventually you will feel some muscle discomfort and tire easily because the minerals used to generate nerve impulses are greatly reduced. You body is running low on electrolytes (natural batteries).

Chapter 7

Neutral Water

Neutral water contains both types of minerals, acidic and alkaline. It is the most natural form of water. Examples of water that have neutral pH include water from the river, sea, and wells. Neutral water is usually obtained near low areas where the altitude is close to sea level.

Although neutral mineral water is the most natural form of water, it cannot help to neutralize the acidic toxic waste in your body. Simple science tells us that we can never neutralize acidity with something neutral. Only water with high alkalinity can neutralize the acidity in your body.

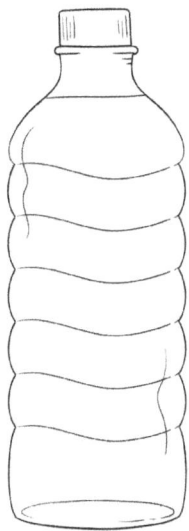

Figure 7.1 Bottled mineral water

The most common source of natural mineral water in the urbanized world is the bottled mineral water sold in the supermarket. If you are lucky, maybe you can find a brand of mineral water that draws water from a source that contains more alkaline minerals that give it some alkalinity.

How About the Tap Water in the Kitchen?

Water that comes from the tap above your kitchen sink is neutral too. This is because the original source of your household water supply is most often the local river. The water has been treated in a water processing plant so that it is clean and safe for household usage.

In the water processing plant, after all the mechanical filtering stages, chlorine is added to kill the bacteria and other microbes found in the water. Now your water might look clean and safe to drink, but what do you know about the potential threat of chlorine?

In the olden days, when our ancestors had to take water from the river or a well for drinking, the only way to kill off the harmful bacteria was by boiling and then letting it cool before drinking it.

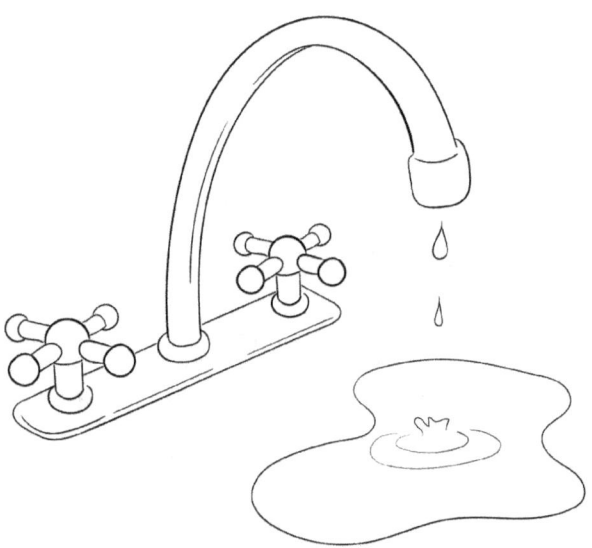

Figure 7.2 Tap water

Now, fast forward to the modern world where clean and chlorinated municipal water is readily available. Some families still practice the boiling and cooling method to prepare drinking water. And most of us still boil water for making tea or coffee.

But there is a problem with boiling water that contains chlorine. When the chlorine in the water is heated to the boiling point, it reacts with certain chemical compounds in the water to form trihalomethane. This compound is a proven carcinogenic, meaning it is one of the substances that can cause cancer.

Furthermore, boiled water is known as "dead water" because it has lost all of its dissolved oxygen content. If you doubt this, try putting a fish into a small aquarium with boiled mineral water and another fish into a same size aquarium containing unboiled water. Observe the movement of both fish over the next 60 minutes, and you will know which type of water is more life sustaining.

Chapter 8

Alkaline Water

In nature, alkaline water is found near mountainous areas where some sources of water gush out from the cracks in the rocks. Some scientific studies have shown that people living around those natural sources of alkaline water tend to live healthier and longer.

Where to Get Alkaline Water?

As more and more good news spreads about the health benefits of drinking alkaline water, people are starting to wonder what is so special about this water. Sadly, few official books or reports provide an unbiased explanation about alkaline water.

You might have read some articles that criticize alkaline water as "snake oil on tap" or some marketing scam. Moreover, those critics also claim that they are chemistry professors or medical doctors. This further adds to the confusion for those regular people trying to find some reliable information on this subject using the Internet.

Searching online, it seems one finds either some extreme critics or commercially biased sales pitches about alkaline water. Here are some neutral facts about different types of alkaline water available in the market and the methods used to produce them.

Alkaline Drops

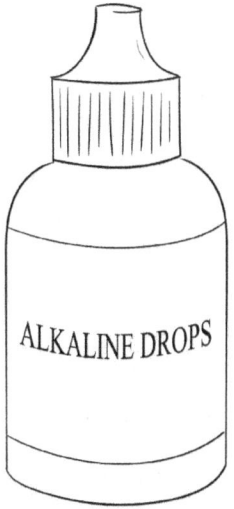

Figure 8.1 Alkaline drops

Alkaline drops (**Figure 8.1**) is actually a concentrated alkaline-mineral solution that can turn a glass of normal water alkaline with just one or two drops. The salesperson claims that this liquid is produced with very advanced technology. All sorts of scientific terms will start to gush from her mouth: "nanotechnology," "hydrogen bomb," "atomic reactions."

I call this a smoke screen sales pitch because it makes you so confused with its scientific mumbo-jumbo that you believe this product actually is very high tech; thus you pay a high price for a tiny bottle of concentrated mineral water.

Alkaline Stick

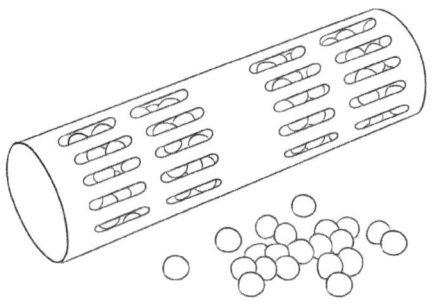

Figure 8.2 Alkaline stick

This is a metal or plastic stick (**Figure 8.2**) full of tiny holes. Inside this alkaline stick are some alkaline minerals stones or beads. All you have to do is to add one or two alkaline sticks to a bottle full of drinking water and ... presto! It becomes alkaline water!

The science behind it is very simple. When you submerge this alkaline stick in your normal drinking water, the minerals inside the stones dissolve in the water and change the pH to slightly alkaline. At first, the alkalinity is very high when the stick is used to treat your water. But after several uses, the alkalinity of the water decreases because most of the alkaline minerals within the stones have been diluted.

Alkaline Flask or Pot

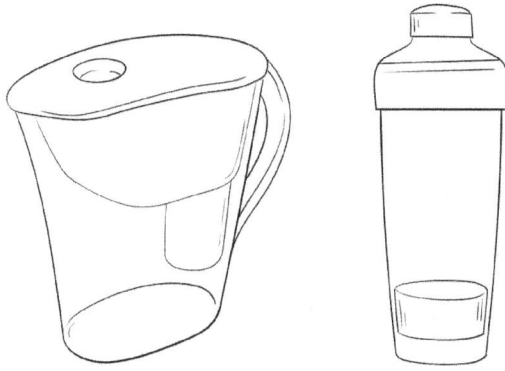

Figure 8.3 Alkaline flasks

This is the newer, repackaged version of the alkaline stick. This "new technology" has become very popular recently, thanks to the active promotion of some MLM companies.

An alkaline flask (**Figure 8.3**) is a thermos-like water flask made of stainless steel and high-quality plastics. Companies claim this magic pot can turn normal water into alkaline and energized water when the water is stored in it for a few hours.

Actually, there is nothing special about this pot. But the special layer of mineral stones added inside the flask gives the alkalizing ability to the product. Those added stones contain some alkaline minerals. Your normal water will turn alkaline when some of those alkaline minerals dissolve.

If fact, you can get effects similar to the alkaline stick or alkaline flask by crushing some dried seashells and putting them in a normal jar or flask and letting it stand for about 15 minutes. You will get a glassful of mildly alkaline water, the same as that produced by those stone-lined flasks. What's the difference? Seashells are free, whereas a stone-lined alkaline flask is expensive.

The reason I said the above methods of producing alkaline water are expensive is because, over time, they are just that. All of them give just a temporary supply of minerals. The fundamental concept they use to produce alkaline water is by adding alkaline minerals to the water. Once that small bottle of alkaline drops is emptied, or the mineral stones no longer contain alkaline minerals, you will not get any more alkalinity until you buy the replacements.

Another huge shortcoming of this type of alkaline water is the alkaline minerals are neither ionized nor activated. Remember, you need the antioxidative effect of negatively charged ions to combat the free radicals in your body.

You might think that the cost of these small items is affordable for you. What about your family members? They need to drink healthy water as much as you do. Go ahead and calculate the total cost for producing alkaline water for your entire family using sticks, drops, and flasks. But don't be surprised to find out that it is going to cost you thousands of dollars a year! You are an MLM salesperson's ideal prospect, so be forewarned.

Hopefully, you can now see why you should seriously consider getting a good alkaline water ionizer unit, which I'm going to discuss in the coming chapter. For your family's long-term health and to permanently say good-bye to your gout, ionized alkaline water is a must.

Chapter 9

Ionized Alkaline Water

Ionized alkaline water is far different from the alkaline water mentioned in the previous chapter. Alkaline drops, alkaline sticks, and alkaline flasks produce alkaline water by utilizing the mineral-addition concept. They cannot produce alkaline water anymore once the alkaline minerals are exhausted.

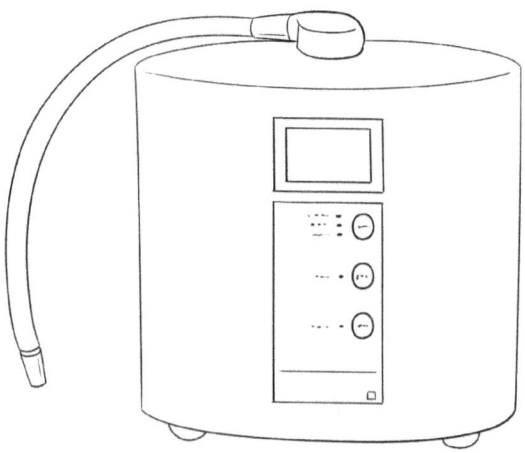

Figure 9.1 Alkaline water ionizer

Ionized alkaline water is a product of the advanced technology used in alkaline water ionizers. The scientific methodology utilized by this machine is actually the opposite of those products mentioned in the previous chapter. An alkaline water ionizer uses dynamic electrolysis technology to separate the existing minerals in the municipal water supply that comes out of your kitchen tap. The fundamental scientific concept behind producing ionized alkaline water using dynamic electrolysis is known as *mineral separation.*

Ionized alkaline water produced using mineral-separation technology is charged with high antioxidative potential, has high alkalinity, and contains much less acidic mineral content than water produced with other methods.

You don't have to study how the electronics inside the alkaline water ionizer works. All you need to know is the fundamental idea of how the ionized alkaline water is produced and how it can help to reverse the hyperuricemia problem you are currently suffering.

Static Electrolysis

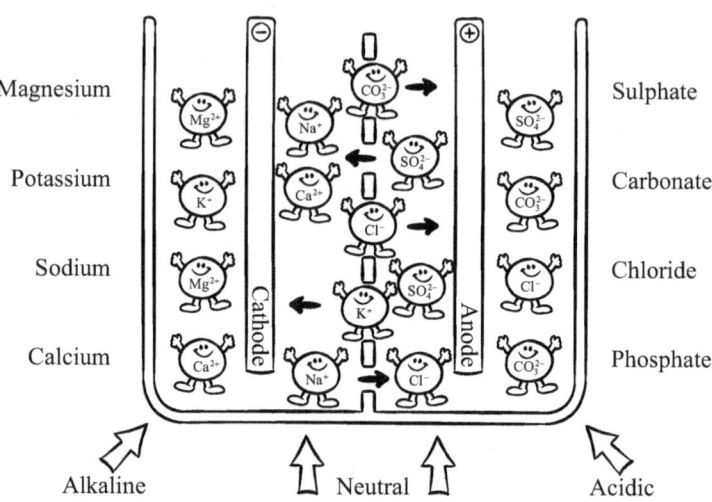

Static Electrolysis

Magnesium	Sulphate
Potassium	Carbonate
Sodium	Chloride
Calcium	Phosphate

Alkaline   Neutral   Acidic

Figure 9.2 Static electrolysis technology

Inside a simplified electrolysis unit, as shown in **Figure 9.2**, are two compartments with electrodes of opposite polarity. Positive alkaline ions near the positive electrode (anode) move toward the negative electrode (cathode) while negative acidic ions near the cathode travel to the opposite side. This happens because the positive electrode repels positive charges and the negative electrode attracts positive charges and vice versa.

The result of this electrical reaction is the separation and concentration of alkaline minerals and acidic minerals. Alkaline water has higher concentrations of alkaline mineral ions; hence potassium, magnesium, calcium, and sodium are present in it. On the other hand, acidic water contains more acidic minerals, such as chlorine, fluorine, lead, sulfur, and phosphorus.

Dynamic Electrolysis

The previous example showed a simplified static electrolysis cell that I used to explain how electrolysis occurs. **Figure 9.3** shows the actual dynamic electrolysis process that happens inside the electrolysis chamber of an alkaline water ionizer.

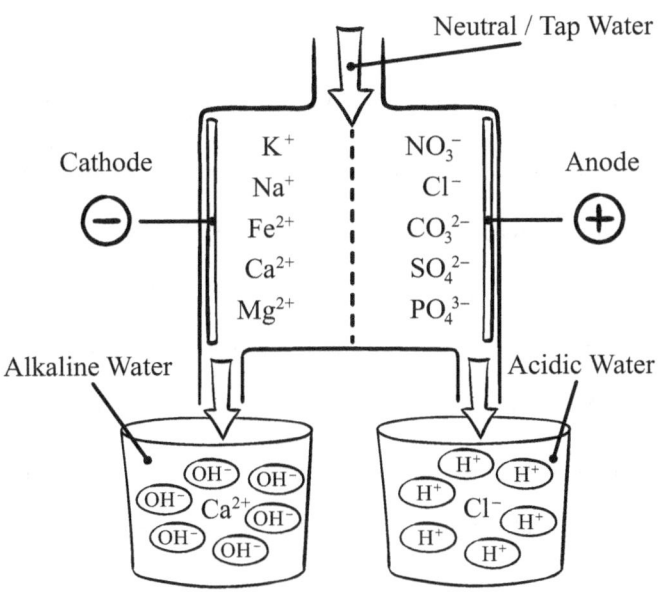

Figure 9.3 Dynamic electrolysis technology

Naturally, a water molecule has the tendency to dissociate or ionize itself into hydrogen ions and hydroxide ions.

$$H2O \rightleftharpoons H^+ \text{ (hydrogen)} + OH^- \text{ (hydroxide)}$$

There is higher concentration of alkaline minerals with positive charges in the water that comes out on the cathode side. These alkaline ions have a strong positive electrostatic charge that attracts hydroxides (H^+), producing ionized alkaline water. Whereas on the anode side, the strong negative electrostatic charge of the acidic mineral ions attracts hydrogen ions and produces ionized acidic water.

It is not the objective of this book to discuss all the technicalities of this ionizer technology. If you want to find out more about this, make sure you subscribe to my newsletter for more future updates.

What Are the Benefits of Ionized Alkaline Water?

There are four unique qualities of ionized alkaline water that other water filtration machines can never produce. It is these four pillars of alkaline water that have helped cure thousands of gout patients.

Here is a brief explanation of the four pillars and how they work:

1. High alkalinity: I believe you have already read enough about the impact of accumulated acidic compounds in your body. And basic science tells us that drinking water with high alkalinity can neutralize the acidity in your body. Almost everyone can see a definite and obvious improvement in their gout condition after drinking alkaline water for a few weeks. Pharmaceuticals don't do this.

2. High negative ORP: ORP stands for oxidation-reduction potential. All chemical reactions, including those that happen inside every cell of your body, involve oxidation and reduction. Free radicals inside your body have positive ORP and act as active oxidation agents; they attack your cells every day and cause your body to age. Not only that, oxidation inside your body is already a proven cause of various illnesses, such as hypertension, gout, and cancer. Ionized alkaline water has high concentrations of hydroxide ions (OH–), which have a high negative ORP. Hydroxide is a good reduction agent that can react with the free radicals in our bodies to "tame" them down. In short, ionized alkaline water has high antioxidation ability; some people even call it an antiaging factor.

3. Smallest molecule cluster: The dynamic electrolysis that produces ionized alkaline water breaks down the water molecule clusters into the smallest size possible. This is critically important: tiny ionized alkaline water molecule clusters can be easily absorbed and expelled from your body cells. In turn, this makes the blood flow better, delivering essential nutrients and removing toxic wastes.

4. The ability to emulsify oil or fat: Because of the fine molecule cluster and the ionized properties of ionized alkaline water, it has the ability to penetrate the oil or fat chemical structure. Thus long-term drinking of alkaline water can help the recovery of hypertension, heart disease, and other fat-related health problems.

Each of the four qualities of ionized alkaline water can be shown clearly with some simple demonstrations. This is pure science, not magic tricks.

Chapter 10

How Ionized Alkaline Water Reverses Hyperuricemia

The intense pain of a gout attack is caused by the inflammation triggered by the urate crystals. There are two different stages of the problem. The short-term problem is the painful gouty inflammation; the long-term problem is the hidden urate crystals. Your objective is to get rid of the long-term problem, but it takes time to dissolve and flush away the uric acid from the affected joint. If you want to get rid of the intense pain fast, deal with the inflammation first, and the most effective way is with the help of NSAIDs.

To deal with the urate crystals, you must first have a clear picture of the pathway of the uric acid accumulation in your body. The excess uric acid is the direct result of your diet habits over the years. The high-purine, protein-rich foods you have eaten have increased the uric acid in the blood plasma, which seeps into the interstitial fluid before ending up being stored in the synovial fluid.

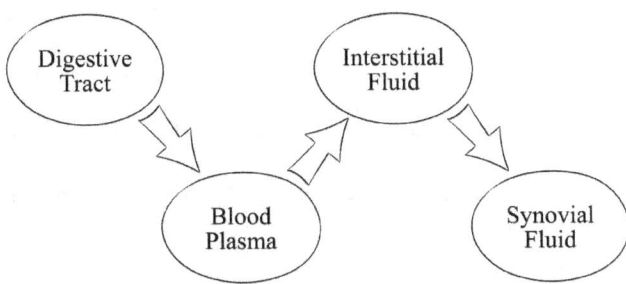

Figure 10.1 Pathway of high-purine, protein-rich foods

It took years for those acidic wastes to seep all the way deep into the synovial fluids of the joints in your body. Ionized alkaline water has to follow the same pathway to track down those acidic compounds and neutralize them.

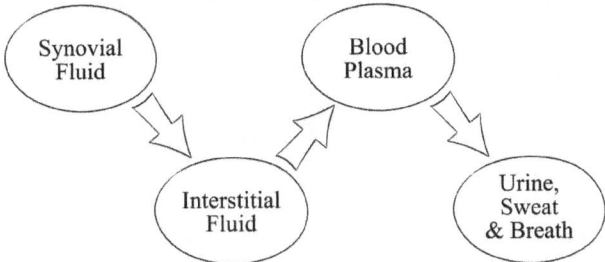

Figure 10.2 Pathway of ionized alkaline water to neutralize acidic waste

The good news is that it is going to take a much shorter time for ionized alkaline water to reverse the process, thanks to the small molecule cluster and actively charged properties of this active water. This enhanced permeability circulates all around the body to bring in the alkalizing minerals and carry out those neutralized wastes.

In my experience with thousands of gout patients, most of them have experienced obvious and healthy reductions in their blood-borne uric acid level after drinking ionized alkaline water for just one month!

But wait! Don't get too excited right away. The damages that those harmful acidic oxidative wastes have done to your body could have reached deep into the joints. Getting rid of the uric acid in the blood can be very fast and direct, but to actually remove the root of the problem (urate crystals in the joints) is going to take some time.

Maybe your blood uric acid level will return to normal healthy level in just a few months with the help of ionized alkaline water. But do not take things for granted and start eating and drinking like nobody's business. You will have to continue your ionized alkaline water drinking habit as long as you want to clear your body from those toxic wastes and maintain an optimum state of health. This should allow you to continue to enjoy everyday life.

Caution!

Do not expect a glass or two of ionized alkaline water to take away your gout pain instantly. If you are currently suffering from a gout attack, you will have to take colchicine or painkillers to manage the pain.

This process takes time. It has taken 10 or years or longer for those acids to accumulate to the toxic level they possess today. Therefore, you should give yourself at least one or two years to clear them all out with the help of ionized alkaline water.

Healing Crisis

When you drink ionized alkaline water for the first time, chances are that you will go through some minor healing crisis. Different people show different signs of this healing crisis. Here are the explanations for the three most common healing crises that many gout patients experience.

Joint Pains

The most common initial reaction felt by many gout patients during their first few days of drinking ionized alkaline water is joint pain. Some even have complained to me that the pain is even worse than a gout attack!

Whenever your body detects any free-floating urate crystal, it alarms the immune system to react to it. The occurrence of urate crystal is caused by the increase in uric acid concentration, which leads to the formation of new urate crystal. Every gout attack means that new urate crystals have formed. The inflammation cannot remove the urate crystal because it is not organic matter, such as bacteria, that can be eaten by the white blood cells. These urate crystals have deposited within the joint. Have your ever experienced gout attack after you had played intense sports that involve a lot of jumping or kicking? The strong vibrations during the game had stirred up some old urate crystals.

The same process happens if you drink too much strong ionized alkaline water within a short time. Sudden introduction of ionized water with very high alkalinity shocks the body's biochemical equilibrium and chemically awakens the old deposited urate crystals, which leads to gout-like attack.

Don't worry; you can prevent this painful healing crisis by following the methods or dosage of ionized alkaline water discussed in the Quick Start Guide.

Upset Stomach

Your digestive tract is filled with hundreds of types of bacteria. Some are good symbiotic bacteria that help your digestion, whereas others are bad parasites that steal nutrients from your daily diet.

Good bacteria in the small intestine prosper under an alkaline environment, whereas parasitic bacteria love acidic surroundings. One simple way (not an expensive colonoscopy) to know which type of bacteria is more common in your gastrointestinal tract is to note the odor of the gas that you pass (flatulence). If it occurs frequently and has an unbearable stench, then you have an acidic intestinal environment that promotes the growth of unhealthy parasites.

At the beginning of your ionized alkaline water therapy, your digestive tract is the first contact point with the water. The sudden change of pH will disturb the lifestyle of those filthy bacteria or fungi, and there will be a miniwar between the good and bad bacteria, which results in stomachache or possible diarrhea.

You should not worry about that. The discomfort will go away in a day or two; the longest I know of lasted about one week. Eventually, the number of bad bacteria will decrease to a minimum, and you will notice there is less or no more unpleasant odor in the "wind that breaks out."

Rise in Body Heat or Fever

In some cases, people feel their body temperature rise, and it seems as though they have a mild fever during the first few days of their ionized alkaline water regimen. Again, my experience has shown this is a fairly common symptom, typically found among those with very acidic intestinal tracts.

> Most of the biochemical reactions inside your body are exothermic (chemical reaction that releases energy in the form of heat). This is what keeps your body temperature at 37.°C (98.6 °F).

For the first few days of ionized alkaline water therapy, you might feel as though you are experiencing a fever. You sweat easily and frequently even when you are sleeping. Don't panic and run to the kitchen to swallow your usual fever pills. This rise in body temperature happens because the neutralization process between alkaline and acidic minerals is very exothermic; it releases a lot heat. You will feel much better over time as your body readjusts its metabolic rate to accommodate the neutralization process. Keep on drinking ionized alkaline water frequently to replenish the water lost through your breath and sweat.

Quick Start Guide

Ionized Alkaline Water Therapy for Gout

Step 1: Get an Alkaline Water Ionizer Unit

If you haven't installed an alkaline water ionizer yet, seriously consider investing in one as soon as possible. I understand purchasing an alkaline water ionizer might be a financial burden for some people due to the high prices charged for these machines. Good ones cost around USD $2,000.

I realize some of you might think, "What?! With the same amount of money, I can buy the latest 40-inch HD LCD TV, the newest iPhone 4G, and several nice dinners out with my family!"

That exact thought pattern is the culprit that underlies the widespread incidence of modern diseases. Our natural preference toward any activity that gives us instant gratification does not lead us toward good health. Nevertheless, we want something that can satisfy our desires instantly.

Do you think you would still enjoy all those nice things available in this modern world if your foot is amputated due to gout and other hyperuricemia-related complications? By then, even an 80-inch SHD LCD TV plus an iPhone 5G will not make you any happier.

Your Health is Priceless

I'm not here to sell you anything or pitch you to buy any particular brand of ionizer. I speak from my personal experience after meeting and consulting with hundreds of gout, diabetes, and cancer patients.

It's hard for me to explain the kind of misery and pain that the victims of these modern diseases suffer daily. You would have to see it for yourself to witness the incalculable suffering. If you look beyond their surgery scars and their tired faces, you can't help but feel a little of the pain and sorrows that beset them.

Drugs and medicines are just a means of controlling and maintaining the symptoms of these illnesses. Those synthetic chemicals will never cure any disease, as they do not attack the root causes. Any student can follow my argument on this.

The logic behind how ionized alkaline water rids you of the root cause of your gout is, to me, obvious, simple, and proven. You don't need all those complex medical terminologies to further obfuscate your problem.

All you need is just one simple answer. And that answer is ionized alkaline water.

Which Brand or Model of Alkaline Water Ionizer Is the Best?

Honestly, I don't have a definite answer to that question. You will come across many websites of different vendors claiming how good their ionizers are compared to other brands. You may be stressed out and confused by all the comparison charts that pop up as you look online for a good alkaline water ionizer.

Focus on what matters. That is my only piece of advice to you regarding which ionizer to choose. As long as the alkaline water ionizer uses reliable electrolysis plates (these must be titanium-platinum), then it is fine. Actually, almost all of the brands/models available in the market are now using titanium-platinum plates.

The main feature that differentiates the better machines is not their pricing, but the quality of their customer service. And that can be a very subjective issue. Contact some of the companies directly, and you will quickly find out their level of professionalism through your conversations.

Don't spend too much time deciding on which one to choose. You might end up with paralysis by analysis and eventually forget about your initial purpose. All you need is an ionizer that can produce clean and safe ionized alkaline water to help you combat hyperuricemia.

Try This

Give yourself three days to do the research and then make the buying decision. If you have found my website and bought this e-book through the recommendation of a friend or relative, and he is already using an alkaline water ionizer at home, then seek his suggestion.

Once the alkaline water ionizer is installed and working properly, then you can begin the course of ionized alkaline water therapy for gout.

Step 2: Follow Through on the Course of Therapy

Depending on the condition of your gout and its complications, you will quite possibly experience a healing crisis during the early stages of your ionized alkaline water therapy. It can be annoying and stressful for some. So, to minimize the impact of this healing crisis, I have come out with the course of a healing crisis for your reference (chart following).

This schedule is based on my observations and feedback from many gout patients. The basic idea here is to gradually increase the neutralization process in your body so that the impact of the healing crisis is softened.

Course of a Healing Crisis		
	pH Level	**Daily Water to Drink**
Day 1–Day 10	Low level (pH ~ 8.5)	2.0 liters ~ 70 ounces
Day 11–Day 30	Mid level (pH ~ 9.5)	3.0 liters ~ 100 ounces

Day 30–onward	High level (pH ~ 10.5 and above)	3.0 liters ~ 100 ounces or more

I know some of you will have concerns about "overalkalinity" or disturbances of your gastric acid from continued drinking of ionized alkaline water that has a very high pH. Please don't worry about this. Long-term drinking of ionized alkaline water will not cause these problems. If it did, I wouldn't be writing this book now.

It is not the scope of this book to explain the biochemical details of overalkalinity and other ionized alkaline-water-related myths as stated on some skeptical websites, such as the "Snake Oil on Tap" by a certain Canadian professor.

Ionized alkaline water works best when consumed on an empty stomach. The best time to take it is in the morning right after waking up and about two hours before or after your evening meal.

Warning!

Do not rush! You must gradually cultivate the water-drinking habit. Give your body enough time to be flexible, to readjust its metabolic rate, and to flush out the acidic waste that has flooded your body's cells for years.

I have seen cases of gout patients not following the recommended way when starting the ionized alkaline water therapy. They wanted fast results. They drank in a few liters of high pH ionized alkaline water over a few hours hoping to get rid of their gout problem quickly. They ended up suffering from various kinds of healing crises.

Get a new calendar on which you write down your targeted daily consumption of ionized alkaline water. Then follow through. If you can, record the total daily volume of ionized alkaline water you drink so you can monitor your consumption.

Step 3: Track Your Progress

Because no one is going to be there to monitor your progress, you are on your own. I strongly suggest you prepare a systematic schedule to record some of the vital figures that reflect the health condition of your internal environment. Kindly refer to the progress record following. You can print it out or create your own Excel spreadsheet file on your computer.

You don't need to prick your finger every day to find out the uric acid level in your blood. Depending on your condition, you can schedule to collect the data (uric acid level and weight) every one or two months.

For gout patients, uric acid level and weight are the vital figures most closely related to gout conditions. Whereas all other data—such as glucose, cholesterol, and blood pressure levels—are for future reference purposes.

Once all those figures fall back into the healthy range, you can show those reports to your doctor and tell her that you don't need her consultation and drugs anymore.

Ionized Alkaline Water Therapy Progress Record						
Day	Date	Weight	Glucose	Uric Acid	Cholesterol	Blood Pressure

Final Words

Congratulations for taking the time to read this far in my book. I hope what I have shared does help you to better understand gout and have a fundamental understanding of ionized alkaline water.

Ionized alkaline water may be something very new to you. It is completely OK and normal to feel skeptical about ionized water as a therapy for a disease that has been around for centuries with no cure.

No one can convince you better than you can. The only way to find out if ionized alkaline water works is to try it for at least three months. Anyway, it is just water that is clear, clean, and safe for drinking. It is many times simpler and safer than those high-tech pharmaceutical drugs.

When you try to solve a complex mathematics problem, do you make it more complex by adding more variables? Of course not! The only way to solve a complicated equation is to rule out all the unnecessary variables and simplify it until only one unknown is left; then you solve the problem. And ionized alkaline water is the simple and effective solution to your complex gout problem.

Conventional medicine is like trying to assemble the pieces of a jigsaw puzzle without actually seeing the picture. It is full of trials and errors, and it is going to be a never-ending process.

Now you have been given a blueprint of the gout problem and have been presented with a logical and proven solution to this predicament of hyperuricemia, all you need to do is give yourself a chance to follow through with the drinking water program.

Don't Take It for Granted

The purpose of going through ionized alkaline water therapy is to rinse out the toxic waste that has accumulated for years. It should not be taken as an antidote or a protective shield against any high-purine or high-protein food diet.

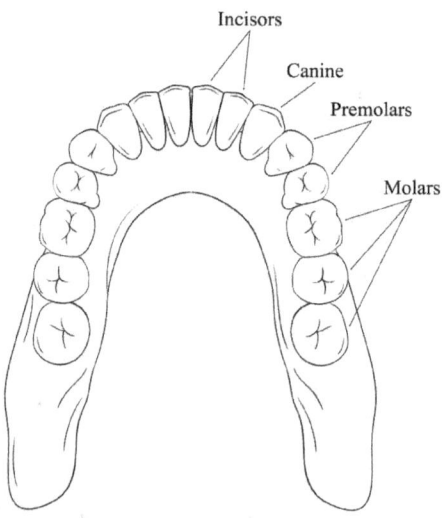

Ionized alkaline water is not a replacement for vegetables. You still need to eat plenty of greens and maintain a well-balanced diet. The perfect ratio is 12.5% meaty protein food and 87.5% plant–based food. Why is this? Well, consider for a minute your teeth. God gives us 32 teeth, 28 are flat (herbivorous) and only 4 are sharp canines (carnivorous). Therefore, 28/32 x 100% = 87.5%.

Not only our teeth but also our digestive tract is at least 80% herbivorous. We are born to eat more plant-based food than meat and other proteins. Our body often cannot digest those excess high-protein foods.

Millions of years of evolution or natural selection have created the physical characteristics that humans now share. But in the past 200 years, our environment has changed many times faster than what our natural process of evolution can keep pace with. It's your choice to be in harmony with the nature of your body or not.

Remember to Check Your E-mail Inbox

More gout and ionized alkaline-water-related topics will be discussed in my upcoming newsletter. Kindly subscribe to the newsletter at www.goutdemystified.com

Should you have any question about ionized alkaline water or gout, kindly write to me at hemen@goutdemystified.com. I will be more than happy to hear your good news or testimony after you've successfully gotten rid of your gout problem.

Last but not least, I would like to wish you and your family great health and to live happily all the time!

Say good-bye to your gout!

Yours sincerely,

Hemen Ee

www.GoutDemystified.com

www.ingramcontent.com/pod-product-compliance
Lightning Source LLC
Chambersburg PA
CBHW070400290526
45790CB00004B/1569